NAVIGATING GAUCHER DISEASE WITH CONFIDENCE AND CARE

Mastering The Journey And Empowering Strategies For Quick Approach To Cancer Healing For Healthy Living

DR. WESLEY IAN

DISCLAIMER

The information in this book is not meant to replace professional medical advice, diagnosis, or treatment; rather, it is meant mainly for general informational reasons. If you have any questions about a medical problem, you should always consult your doctor or another trained health expert. Don't ever discount expert medical advice or put off getting it because of something you've read in this book.

Any negative effects or repercussions arising from the usage of the material provided herein are not the responsibility of the book's author or publisher. It should be noted by readers that the material in this book is not all-inclusive and might not address every facet of the subject. Furthermore, new research may have an impact on how health concerns are understood or treated because medical knowledge is always changing.

No particular test, treatment, method, or product mentioned in this book is endorsed or promoted by the author or publisher. The reader assumes all risk associated with using the information included in this book.

Before making any big decisions regarding your health, it's crucial to speak with a licensed healthcare provider. The relationship between a patient and their healthcare practitioner should not be replaced by this book, nor is it meant to offer medical advice.

The opinions presented in this book are the author's and may not necessarily represent those of the publisher. Any errors, omissions, or inaccuracies in the information in this book are not the responsibility of the author or publisher.

It is recommended that readers independently confirm any information contained in this book and speak with a healthcare provider about their specific medical needs and state of health.

TABLE OF CONTENTS

ABOUT THE BOOK

For people and families impacted by Gaucher Disease, "Navigating Gaucher Disease with Confidence and Care" is an excellent resource that provides a thorough manual for comprehending, coping with, and thriving despite the difficulties connected to this uncommon genetic illness. An intelligent introduction to the book sets the ground for a full examination of Gaucher's Disease. To ensure that readers have a basic understanding of Gaucher Disease, the first few chapters offer a thorough explanation and overview, explaining the different forms of the disorder and exploring its genetic foundations.

Concentrates on the essential elements of diagnosing and comprehending symptoms. Through early detection of symptoms and testing procedures, the book provides readers with the necessary knowledge to manage the intricacies of Gaucher's Disease. It also offers helpful advice on how to live with Gaucher, detailing the expectations that sufferers and their families should have for the duration of the trip.

The book's examination of therapy choices is one of its strongest points. Readers are better equipped to make decisions regarding their healthcare thanks to the thorough analysis of developing medicines, substrate reduction therapy (SRT), and enzyme replacement therapy (ERT). By offering a comprehensive picture of the range of treatment options, the inclusion of complementary and alternative techniques enhances the conversation even more.

The treatment of Gaucher Disease symptoms and consequences is covered in detail. From organ involvement and hematologic difficulties to bone health and osteoporosis, the book offers helpful guidance for managing the various issues that people may confront.

The focus shifts to lifestyle and nutrition, with specific advice on what to eat, how much exercise to get, and mental health. The holistic approach to well-being places a strong emphasis on how crucial a balanced lifestyle is to the successful management of Gaucher Disease.

Navigating day-to-day problems takes center stage. Topics covered include managing pain, overcoming exhaustion, preserving independence, and creating a support network. The book acknowledges the wider effects of Gaucher Disease on day-to-day living in addition to its medical elements.

A comprehensive overview of family planning, education, employment, travel, and leisure is provided. The book provides helpful guidance for people and families on a variety of topics, including genetic counseling, pregnancy issues, and navigating adjustments at work and school. To guarantee thorough support, it also emphasizes how important it is to establish relationships with patient organizations and advocacy groups as well as to make use of financial and insurance resources.

"Navigating Gaucher Disease with Confidence and Care" is an extensive manual that covers the practical, emotional, and social aspects of living with Gaucher Disease in addition to medical knowledge.

CHAPTER ONE

INTRODUCTION TO GAUCHER DISEASE

DEFINITION AND SYNOPSIS

Under the category of lysosomal storage diseases, Gaucher Disease is an uncommon genetic disorder that impairs the body's capacity to metabolize glucocerebroside, a particular class of lipid molecule. Gaucher Disease, so named in honor of the French physician Philippe Gaucher, who originally reported the illness in 1882, is caused by mutations in the GBA gene that result in a glucocerebrosidase enzyme deficiency. This enzyme is essential for the breakdown of glucocerebroside in lysosomes, which are cellular organelles that eliminate waste.

As such, the build-up of unprocessed glucocerebroside within cells might result in various signs and issues.

GAUCHER DISEASE TYPES

Fundamentally, glucocerebroside accumulates abnormally in the spleen, liver, and bone marrow, which is the hallmark of Gaucher Disease. Three primary kinds of the disease are distinguished from its varied clinical presentations: Type 1, Type 2, and Type 3. The most common type, type 1, is identified by its non-neurological symptoms, such as anemia, abnormalities of the bones, and hepatosplenomegaly (enlargement of the liver and spleen). On the other hand, Types 2 and 3 involve neurological issues. Type 3 is a more chronic and progressive form that may appear in childhood or adolescence, while Type 2 is an acute and severe form that frequently presents in infancy and progresses quickly.

FACTORS AND HEREDITY

Comprehending the genesis of Gaucher Disease requires an understanding of its genetic foundations. Due to the primary autosomal recessive inheritance pattern of the disorder, an individual has to inherit two mutant copies of the GBA gene, one from each parent, to become ill. The enzyme glucocerebrosidase is encoded by the GBA gene, which is found on chromosome 1. Mutations in both copies of the GBA gene cause a deficiency in functional glucocerebrosidase in people with Gaucher Disease, which causes glucocerebroside to build up in cells.

Gaucher Disease is complicated due to several issues, such as the wide variety of GBA gene mutations and how they affect the action of enzymes. While some mutations result in lesser symptoms, others may cause more severe forms of the disease. An extra layer of complexity to the comprehension of Gaucher Disease is the non-trivial nature of the link between genotype and phenotype in this condition.

Gaucher Disease is a complex genetic illness with varying clinical manifestations and underlying genetic complexities. Its effects on those who are afflicted can vary from mild neurological symptoms to serious neurological problems.

The disease's genetic basis highlights the importance of familial considerations in its diagnosis and management, while ongoing research continues to deepen our understanding of the diverse mutations associated with Gaucher Disease, paving the way for targeted therapies and improved patient outcomes.

CHAPTER TWO
RECOGNIZING AND INTERPRETING SYMPTOMS
IDENTIFYING THE FIRST SYMPTOMS AND SIGNS

Early detection of signs and symptoms is essential for prompt diagnosis and successful treatment of a variety of illnesses, including but not limited to hereditary disorders such as Gaucher disease. Prompt intervention is made possible by early detection, which may reduce complications and enhance overall prognosis. Early symptoms of Gaucher disease, an inherited condition brought on by a lack of the glucocerebrosidase enzyme, can include easy bruising, inexplicable weariness, and an enlarged liver or spleen. Both patients and medical professionals should be on the lookout for these small but important signs.

Furthermore, being aware of the various ways a given ailment can show itself is necessary to recognize early indicators. For example, there are various forms of

Gaucher disease, each with unique symptoms and rates of progression. The most prevalent type, type 1, can cause symptoms like anemia, bone discomfort, and a higher risk of fractures. But in addition to the more common physical symptoms, Type 2 and Type 3 may also involve neurological issues. Early symptom differentiation and recognition can be improved for healthcare practitioners by raising awareness of the many forms of Gaucher's illness.

PROCEDURES FOR DIAGNOSIS

For disease management to be effective, accurate diagnosis is essential. Diagnostic methods are crucial in validating concerns sparked by observed symptoms in the context of Gaucher's illness. The two main methods used to diagnose Gaucher's disease are genetic testing and blood tests that measure the activity of the glucocerebrosidase enzyme. These examinations support the construction of a customized treatment plan by assisting in the identification of the disorder's presence as well as its precise type and degree.

Gaucher disease-related bone abnormalities can be evaluated with imaging procedures like magnetic resonance imaging (MRI) and X-rays. A characteristic feature of the illness is skeletal involvement, and diagnostic imaging helps to provide a thorough picture of the degree of bone loss. Furthermore, tracking the growth of an organ using imaging methods such as computed tomography (CT) scans or ultrasound helps assess the course of the disease and guide treatment choices.

GAUCHER LIVING: WHAT TO ANTICIPATE

Living with Gaucher's illness requires a multifaceted approach that includes emotional and social factors in addition to medical therapy. Patients with Gaucher disease and those who care for them should plan routine check-ups to assess the efficacy of enzyme replacement therapy (ERT), control symptoms, and handle any consequences. Sustaining a decent quality of life and achieving the best possible health results depend on following through on prescribed treatments and drugs.

In addition, people might have to modify their lifestyles to meet the demands of Gaucher's illness. This could entail changing one's diet, exercising in moderation, and developing pain and tiredness management techniques. To assist people in dealing with the psychological and social effects of having a chronic illness, emotional support from family, friends, and medical professionals is equally important.

A thorough and proactive approach to managing this complicated genetic ailment involves identifying early indications and symptoms, getting the right diagnosis, and adjusting to living with Gaucher disease. With appropriate intervention, comprehensive care, and informed knowledge, people with Gaucher disease can travel through life with increased resilience and well-being.

CHAPTER THREE

OPTIONS FOR TREATMENT

TREATMENT WITH ENZYME REPLACEMENT (ERT)

One therapeutic strategy used to treat certain genetic illnesses, especially lysosomal storage diseases, is called enzyme replacement therapy, or ERT. These disorders result from defects in particular enzymes that break down different chemicals in lysosomes, which are cellular waste disposal organs. To make up for the lack or malfunctioning of endogenous enzymes, exogenous enzyme therapy, or ERT, is used. The goals of this treatment are to lessen symptoms, stop the disease from getting worse, and enhance the quality of life for those who are impacted.

ERT is frequently used to treat illnesses like Pompe disease, Fabry disease, and Gaucher disease. Regular intravenous infusions of the absent enzyme are usually part of the therapy, which helps the damaged organs function better by clearing accumulated substrates. It's vital to remember that although ERT has shown promise in treating symptoms, the underlying genetic abnormality may not entirely improve. To maintain therapeutic results, dosing must frequently be consistent and ongoing.

TREATMENT FOR SUBSTANCE REDUCTION (SRT)

A further therapeutic approach used in the treatment of some hereditary illnesses, including sphingolipidoses, is called substrate reduction therapy (SRT). These conditions are characterized by the aberrant build-up of particular substrates—like sphingolipids—in cells as a result of insufficiencies in the enzymes that break them down. By lowering the synthesis of these substrates, SRT seeks to impede the disease's development.

In contrast to ERT, which uses enzyme supplements to make up for deficiencies, SRT uses tiny compounds to prevent the creation of accumulating substrates. This method assists in addressing the disease's cellular etiology. Conditions such as Niemann-Pick disease and Gaucher disease are treated with SRT. SRT has shown promise in helping to improve some symptoms and delay the progression of certain diseases, even though it might not be able to completely cure them.

NEW THERAPIES

Treatment options for genetic illnesses are constantly changing as new therapeutic techniques are developed as a result of continuing research and development. A wide variety of techniques are included in emerging medicines, such as gene therapy, mRNA-based therapeutics, and small molecule medications that target particular biological processes.

To fix the underlying genetic problem, functioning genes are inserted into the patient's cells through gene therapy. This strategy has been effective in preclinical and early clinical trials and has promise for treating the underlying causes of genetic diseases. Targeting gene expression at the RNA level, mRNA-based therapies—like RNA interference (RNAi)—offer a potentially reversible and focused means of treating genetic diseases.

Research is also being done on small-molecule medications that are intended to target particular cellular pathways connected to the pathophysiology of disease. When compared to conventional methods, these substances might provide alternate therapy choices with possibly fewer adverse effects. Future treatments for genetic illnesses could be more accurate and effective thanks to the field of emerging therapeutics.

ALTERNATIVE AND COMPLEMENTARY METHODS

In addition to traditional medicines, complementary and alternative approaches are frequently employed to enhance the overall care of genetic disorders. These methods cover a wide range of interventions, such as mind-body techniques, acupuncture, herbal therapies, nutritional supplements, and dietary changes.

Complementary and alternative therapies can help reduce symptoms, enhance the efficacy of primary treatment modalities, and improve overall well-being in the setting of genetic illnesses. For instance, to address specific nutritional deficiencies linked to particular hereditary diseases, dietary adjustments, and nutritional supplements may be advised. Furthermore, techniques like yoga and meditation can help people with genetic illnesses manage their stress and enhance their mental health.

It is important to proceed cautiously while utilizing complementary and alternative therapies, making sure that they are incorporated into a thorough treatment plan under the supervision of medical professionals. These methods are not meant to take the place of accepted medical therapies for genetic illnesses, even if they could help manage symptoms and promote overall well-being. A more thorough and patient-centered care plan may benefit from an integrated and cooperative approach that blends traditional and complementary modalities.

CHAPTER FOUR

HANDLING COMPLICATIONS AND SYMPTOMS

OSTEOPENIA AND BONE HEALTH

For those treating a variety of medical disorders, maintaining optimal bone health is essential. One prevalent concern is osteoporosis, which is characterized by the weakening of the bones and an increased risk of fractures. Age, hormone fluctuations, and specific drugs are among the many causes of this illness. People who suffer from long-term conditions like inflammatory bowel disease or rheumatoid arthritis may be more susceptible to osteoporosis. A variety of techniques are included in management efforts, including as frequent weight-bearing activity, lifestyle changes, and sufficient calcium and vitamin D intake.

Doctors may recommend drugs to patients who already have weakened bones to increase bone density and lower their chance of breaking a bone. Frequent monitoring CHAPTER FIusing bone density scans enables medical practitioners to evaluate the success of therapies and modify treatment regimens accordingly. In addition, it is crucial to provide patients with education that highlights the significance of following recommended treatment plans and making lifestyle modifications to lessen the effects of osteoporosis on general health.

HEMATOLOGIC DISORDERS

Hematologic complications are a broad category of problems that impact blood and its constituent parts, frequently creating difficulties for people who are treating long-term medical disorders. Anemia, thrombocytopenia, and coagulation abnormalities are conditions that may develop as a result of the underlying illness or as an adverse reaction to specific medications. Fatigue and impaired oxygen delivery can result from anemia, which is defined as a low red blood cell count or inadequate hemoglobin. Low platelet counts, or thrombocytopenia, raise the risk of bleeding, and coagulation disorders can cause abnormal blood clotting.

A customized strategy is required for the management of hematologic problems, taking into account the particular blood condition and its underlying causes. Blood transfusions, drugs that increase the formation of red blood cells, and clotting factor regulation are a few examples of this. It is crucial to regularly check blood levels to identify and quickly treat any problems. Comprehensive care also includes teaching patients how to recognize the warning signs of hematologic problems and how to follow their prescribed treatment plans.

ORGAN PARTICIPATION AND ADMINISTRATION

Organ involvement is common in chronic illnesses, so a complete management plan is required to address the underlying condition as well as the effects on individual organs. Diseases such as systemic lupus erythematosus, scleroderma, or diabetes can impair essential organs like the heart, lungs, kidneys, and liver. To track organ function and identify any issues early, routine medical examinations and imaging tests are necessary.

Medication designed to control inflammation and stop additional harm to the afflicted organs may be part of treatment regimens. To maintain organ health, lifestyle adjustments like food adjustments and exercise recommendations may be made in specific circumstances. A comprehensive approach to organ involvement is ensured through collaborative care including a multidisciplinary team of medical specialists, including experts in cardiology, nephrology, and pulmonology.

In organ treatment, patient involvement and education are essential. A proactive approach to health is fostered by empowering people to notice warning indications of organ issues, comprehend their diseases, and follow prescribed therapies. Encouraging dialogue and frequent check-ins between patients and medical staff are key components of efficient organ transplantation and enhanced quality of life overall.

CHAPTER FIVE

CONSUMPTION AND WAY OF LIFE

THE DIETARY GUIDELINES

A person's diet is a major factor in their overall health, and sustaining good health requires making educated food choices. A varied range of nutrients, such as carbs, proteins, fats, vitamins, and minerals, should be included in a balanced diet. A diet rich in nutrients is enhanced by emphasizing entire foods, such as fruits, vegetables, whole grains, and lean proteins. Portion control is essential to avoid overindulging because consuming too many calories can result in weight gain and other health problems.

In addition to macronutrients, micronutrients like vitamins and minerals are important for numerous physiological activities. People are urged to satisfy their dietary requirements by consuming a wide variety of vibrant meals. Reducing the risk of chronic diseases and promoting cardiovascular health requires limiting the consumption of processed foods, added sugars, and harmful fats.

It is essential to tailor dietary advice to each individual depending on criteria including age, gender, activity level, and health issues. Athletes, for example, might need a different nutrient balance than sedentary people, and people with particular medical disorders could need dietary therapies that are specifically designed for them. Another essential component of a balanced diet that promotes optimal body functions and general well-being is drinking enough water.

PHYSICAL ACTIVITY AND EXERCISE

A healthy lifestyle is based on regular physical activity, which promotes mental and physical health. Combining aerobic, strength-training, and flexibility workouts promotes flexibility, increases muscle strength, and preserves cardiovascular health. Strength training exercises should be performed at least twice a week in addition to 150 minutes of moderate-intensity activity per week, according to the American College of Sports Medicine.

Exercise regimens are just one aspect of physical activity; it's also crucial to include movement into everyday activities like walking, using the stairs, and engaging in leisure pursuits. Weight control, a happier mood, better cognitive function, and a lower chance of chronic illnesses like diabetes and heart disease are all advantages of regular exercise.

People should engage in activities they enjoy if they want to maintain an active lifestyle over time. To avoid injuries, it's also critical to take into account one's current level of fitness and go gradually to more strenuous activities. Fitting physical activity with one's tastes and health objectives guarantees that exercise becomes a fun and sustainable aspect of daily life.

WELL-BEING AND MENTAL HEALTH

The need to place a high priority on mental health is highlighted by the complex relationship between mental and physical health. A comprehensive strategy for mental health includes things like social support, mindfulness exercises, appropriate sleep, and stress management. Deep breathing techniques, yoga, and meditation are among the stress-relieving activities that might support resilience and emotional equilibrium.

Maintaining a good work-life balance is essential to avoiding burnout and fostering mental wellness. A healthy sleep schedule is essential for maintaining mental clarity, emotional stability, and general vitality. Creating and sustaining supportive social networks—whether via family, friends, or community involvement—offers a vital safety net that boosts mental toughness.

It is imperative to tackle the stigma around mental health to promote candid discussions and timely assistance. Getting professional help, like therapy or counseling, can be very helpful in managing mental health issues. Understanding the relationship between mental and physical health promotes a more holistic view of health, highlighting the significance of an integrated and balanced lifestyle for general vitality.

CHAPTER SIX
HANDLING DAY-TO-DAY OBSTACLES
HANDLING EXHAUSTION

Among the many difficulties we face daily, managing weariness is one that is prevalent and frequently disregarded. Both physical and mental exhaustion can have a big influence on a person's capacity to perform everyday duties and responsibilities. The secret is to spot the symptoms early and put good fatigue management and relief techniques into practice. Combating weariness requires regular exercise, a healthy diet, and enough sleep. To improve their resilience in the face of fatigue, people could also find benefits in implementing mindfulness techniques like deep breathing exercises or meditation.

PAIN MANAGEMENT

Managing the experience of chronic pain can be a complex task that calls for a multimodal strategy. In addition to taking medicine, managing pain also entails looking into complementary therapies and making lifestyle changes. Physical therapy, acupuncture, and relaxation techniques are just a few of the numerous methods that people might use to reduce pain. Open communication between patients and medical staff is crucial to developing a customized pain management strategy that takes into account each patient's particular circumstances. People can empower themselves to better manage the difficulties of chronic pain by taking a comprehensive approach.

PRESERVING INDEPENDENCE

Keeping one's independence is essential for overcoming obstacles in life, particularly as things change. Whether dealing with cognitive decline, physical restrictions, or other issues that impair autonomy, people can look into several options to keep their sense of freedom. When it comes to encouraging self-sufficiency, assistive technologies, home adaptations, and adaptive methods can make a big difference. In addition, cultivating a resilient and adaptive attitude enables people to deal with changing situations gracefully and maintain their independence in the face of shifting obstacles.

PUTTING TOGETHER A SUPPORT NETWORK

There is no denying that navigating daily obstacles is easier when you have a strong support network. Developing and preserving deep relationships with friends, family, and neighbors provides an essential safety net in trying times. Support networks can provide a feeling of community, practical help, and emotional support. These connections are strengthened by reciprocity and effective communication, which enable people to share the load of difficulties and rejoice in victories with one another. Knowing that there is a solid support system in place can be reassuring and uplifting during trying times, building resilience in the face of life's unavoidable setbacks.

CHAPTER SEVEN

GAUCHER DISEASE AND FAMILY PLANNING

GENETIC COUNSELING

In the context of Gaucher Disease, a rare genetic illness brought on by a glucocerebrosidase enzyme deficiency, genetic counseling is essential. Those with a family history of the disease or who are carriers may wish to consult a genetic counselor to learn about the consequences for both themselves and their future children. Genetic counselors offer details on the disease's inheritance pattern, the possibility of passing it on to subsequent generations, and the many testing alternatives.

Individuals and families are informed about the advantages and disadvantages of genetic testing during genetic counseling sessions. People can use this knowledge to make educated decisions about having children and family planning. To make sure that individuals and couples feel supported in navigating the intricacies connected with Gaucher Disease, the counselor takes into account the emotional and psychological components of the material offered.

GAUCHER DISEASE AND PREGNANCY

Those who have the disease or who carry it must take special precautions during pregnancy. Specialized care may be necessary for women with this illness to maintain their health and the health of the growing fetus. To ascertain whether the unborn child has inherited Gaucher Disease, genetic testing may be made available to expectant parents. With the help of this information, parents may make decisions about their pregnancy and get ready for any obstacles that may arise.

Due to hormonal changes and greater demands on the body, some people with Gaucher Disease may occasionally experience an aggravation of symptoms during pregnancy. To treat any difficulties that may occur during pregnancy, close supervision by a healthcare team of specialists aware of the complexities of Gaucher Disease is necessary. When caring for pregnant patients with Gaucher Disease, medical personnel must balance the mother's health with the possible effects on the fetus.

PARENTING WITH GAUCHER DISEASE

Raising a child with Gaucher Disease necessitates a thorough and interdisciplinary approach. Ongoing assistance and education are beneficial for individuals with the illness and their spouses in managing the obstacles that come with raising a family. Unique challenges that parents may encounter include educating their kids about the nature of Gaucher Disease and responding to any worries or inquiries that may come up.

Maintaining open lines of contact with medical professionals is essential to managing the symptoms and treatment of Gaucher Disease while carrying out the duties of motherhood. Parents have to find a way to balance taking care of their own health needs with giving their kids a loving atmosphere. Support systems, such as patient advocacy groups and counseling programs, can be extremely helpful to families in managing the practical and emotional challenges of raising a child with Gaucher disease.

The relationship between Gaucher Disease and family planning necessitates thoroughly thought-out genetic counseling, difficulties associated with pregnancy, and the dynamics of raising a child with a chronic genetic illness. Individuals and families impacted by Gaucher Disease can manage these complications with resilience and adaptation by adopting a holistic and knowledgeable approach.

CHAPTER EIGHT

EDUCATION AND EMPLOYMENT

MANAGING SCHOOLING WHILE HAVING GAUCHER DISEASE

For those who live with this uncommon genetic illness, navigating school can provide special obstacles. A disorder known as Gaucher Disease is characterized by an accumulation of fatty substances in different organs due to the body's incapacity to break down a particular form of fat.

It takes careful balancing for kids with Gaucher Disease to manage their health and academic aspirations. Building a learning environment involves collaborating with healthcare providers, educational institutions, and support systems.

Proactive communication is vital in the field of education. To discuss their requirements, students with Gaucher Disease should have open communication with educators, administrators, and disability services. This could entail talking about possible concessions like flexible attendance guidelines, longer deadlines, or a peaceful, pleasant area to relax in. Through promoting knowledge and awareness of Gaucher Disease, people can help create a positive learning environment that supports their achievement.

WORKPLACE MODIFICATIONS

When moving from academic to professional settings, workplace accommodations for people with Gaucher Disease are crucial. Employers are essential in fostering an inclusive workplace because they make the required modifications to address the particular difficulties that this condition presents.

This could entail offering flexible work schedules, ergonomic workplaces, or access to on-site medical facilities. Employers can support individuals with Gaucher Disease in thriving in their professional jobs by providing an understanding and supportive work environment.

SPEAKING UP FOR YOURSELF

For people with Gaucher Disease to navigate both education and employment, learning how to advocate for oneself becomes crucial. Self-advocacy is stating one's needs clearly, being aware of one's limits, and proactively pursuing the help one needs. In school contexts, this could entail supporting awareness campaigns to foster understanding among peers and educators and collaborating closely with disability services to guarantee that accommodations are in place.

To negotiate adjustments, people with Gaucher Disease may need to start conversations with human resources departments or managers at work. Creating a culture of support at work can entail educating coworkers about the illness. A more inclusive educational and professional environment can be fostered by individuals with Gaucher Disease by actively engaging in discussions about their needs and raising awareness.

Navigating education and the workplace with Gaucher Disease takes a holistic approach that incorporates open communication, proactive advocacy, and a dedication to creating understanding. People with Gaucher Disease can actively create circumstances that support their academic and professional success by actively interacting with companies and educational institutions. Self-advocacy is still an effective strategy because it gives people the ability to express their needs and make a positive, inclusive community.

CHAPTER NINE

MATERIALS AND ASSISTANCE

PATIENT ASSOCIATIONS AND CAMPAIGN TEAMS

Patient organizations and advocacy groups are essential in helping people with a range of health issues, including those caused by diseases such as Gaucher disease. People with specific medical conditions or those with similar health concerns typically join these organizations. These support groups can provide Gaucher patients with a feeling of belonging, empathy, and common experiences. Patient organizations and advocacy groups are effective means for individuals to come together, exchange knowledge, and fight for better healthcare regulations and initiatives about research on Gaucher disease.

Joining an advocacy group or patient organization gives people access to helpful information and support systems, which is a noteworthy benefit. To stay up to date on the most recent advancements in Gaucher disease research and treatment possibilities, these groups frequently work in conjunction with medical experts, researchers, and pharmaceutical companies. They also provide a forum for patients and their families to exchange personal narratives, coping mechanisms, and guidance, creating a supportive atmosphere that extends beyond the realm of medicine.

GETTING IN TOUCH WITH THE GAUCHER NATION

Establishing connections with patient organizations within the Gaucher community offers a special means of empowerment and emotional support. It might be lonely to have a rare sickness, but these communities' help people connect beyond geographic borders. Online communities, neighborhood support groups, and yearly conferences provide people with a platform to share ideas, talk about difficulties, and commemorate achievements in unison.

These groups improve the general well-being of Gaucher patients and their families by creating a sense of community.

RESOURCES FOR MONEY AND INSURANCE

Resources related to finances and insurance are essential parts of a full package of care for people with Gaucher illness. One typical concern is how to manage the financial load of medical treatments, prescription drugs, and other healthcare bills. To offer advice on managing insurance coverage, gaining access to financial assistance programs, and comprehending available resources, patient organizations and advocacy groups frequently work with financial specialists. With this support, people with Gaucher's illness can concentrate on their health without having undue financial stress.

Additionally, these organizations might actively participate in lobbying campaigns to impact healthcare regulations and encourage greater accessibility to reasonably priced medical care. Patient organizations work together to develop joint projects that not only address the medical elements of Gaucher disease but also promote fair and equal access to resources that improve patient's quality of life in general.

For people and families impacted by Gaucher disease, patient organizations and advocacy groups are vital. Through fostering a sense of community among the Gaucher community, they enable individuals to effectively manage the obstacles associated with their condition. Furthermore, the availability of Financial and Insurance Resources guarantees that pragmatic obstacles, such as financial limitations, do not impede the acquisition of essential healthcare. Together, these factors constitute a complete support network that goes beyond medical care, contributing to the entire well-being of persons touched by Gaucher disease.